AIR FRYER COOKBOOK

FOR BEGINNERS

Cook Truly Healthy and Satisfying Food Effortlessly
Through 37 Easy and Quick Recipes for New Chefs
and Learners.

Philbert Gordon

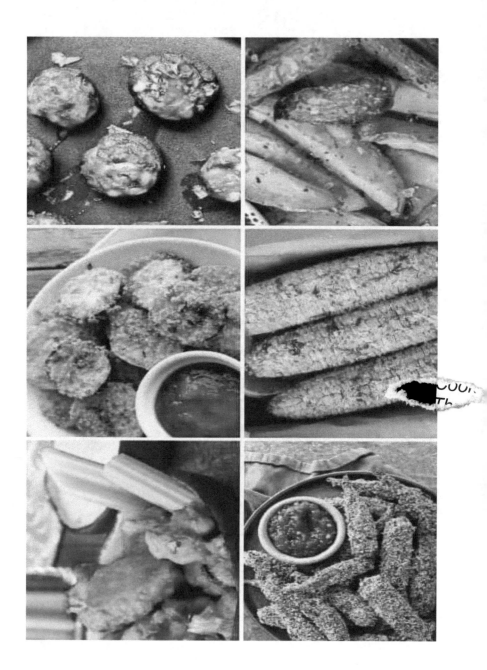

Table of Contents

INTRODUCTION

An air fryer is like an oven as in it prepares and broils, however the thing that matters is its heating components are just situated on top and are joined by a large, incredible fan, bringing about food that is very firm instantly — and, most outstandingly, with less oil than rotisserie partners. Air fryers typically heat up rapidly and they cook food rapidly and equitably, on account of the blend of a concentrated heat source and the size and position of the fan.

Another incredible piece of air browning is the cleanup. Most air fryer bushels and racks are dishwasher safe. For the ones that are not dishwasher safe, we propose a decent dish brush, similar to this one from Casabella.

Air fryers are quick, and once you see how they work, they can be utilized to heat frozen food varieties or cook such new food like chicken, steak, pork hacks, salmon and veggies. Most meats require no additional oil since they're as of now so delicious: simply season them with salt and your #1 spices and flavors. Ensure you stick to dry flavors — less dampness prompts crispier outcomes. In the event that you need to treat meats with grill sauce or nectar, stand by until the two or three minutes of cooking.

Lean cuts of meat, or food sources with practically no fat, expect oil to brown and fresh up. Brush boneless chicken breasts and pork hacks with a touch of oil prior to preparing. Vegetable oil or canola oil is usually prescribed because of its higher smoke point, which means it can tolerate upping to the high heat in an air fryer.

Vegetables likewise should be thrown in oil before air broiling. We suggest sprinkling them with salt before air broiling; yet utilize somewhat less than you're utilized to: The fresh, air singed bits pack a ton of flavor. We love air broiling broccoli florets, Brussels fledglings and child potato parts. They come out so fresh! Butternut squash, yams and beets all appear to get better, and green beans and peppers take no time at all.

Air fryer meals recipes

35+ recipes

1. Air fryer Cauliflower Tots

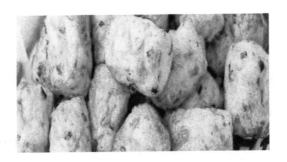

YIELDS: 6 SERVINGS | PREP TIME: 0 HOURS 10 MINS | COOK TIME: 0 HOURS 0 MINS | TOTAL TIME: 0 HOURS 30 MINS

INGREDIENTS

- Cooking splash
- 4 c. cauliflower florets, steamed (around 1/2 huge cauliflower)
- 1 huge egg, daintily beaten
- 1 c. shredded cheddar
- 1 c. newly ground Parmesan
- 2/3 c. panko breadcrumbs
- 2 tbsp. newly chopped chives

- Genuine salt
- Newly ground dark pepper
- 1/2 c. ketchup
- 2 tbsp. Sriracha

DIRECTIONS

FOR OVEN

1. Preheat oven to 375°. Oil a huge preparing sheet with cooking splash.

2. In a food processor, beat steamed cauliflower until rice. Spot riced cauliflower on a perfect kitchen towel and press to deplete water.

3. Move cauliflower to a huge bowl with egg, cheddar, Parmesan, Panko, and chives and blend until consolidated. Season with salt and pepper to taste.

4. Spoon around 1 tablespoon blend and fold it into a potato child shape with your hands. Spot on arranged preparing sheet and heat for 15 to 20 minutes, until toddlers are brilliant.

5. In the interim, make zesty ketchup: Combine ketchup and Sriracha in a little serving bowl and mix to join.

6. Serve warm cauliflower children with fiery ketchup.

FOR AIR FRYER

1. In a food processor, beat steamed cauliflower until rice. Spot riced cauliflower on a perfect kitchen towel and press to deplete water.

2. Move cauliflower to a huge bowl with egg, cheddar, Parmesan, Panko, and chives and blend until joined. Season with salt and pepper to taste.

3. Spoon around 1 tablespoon blend and fold it into a potato toddler shape with your hands. Working in clusters, organize in bin of air fryer in a solitary layer and cook at 375° for 10, until children are brilliant.

4. In the interim, make zesty ketchup: Combine ketchup and Sriracha in a little serving bowl and mix to join.

5. Serve warm cauliflower toddlers with hot ketchup.

2. Air Fryer Brussels Sprouts

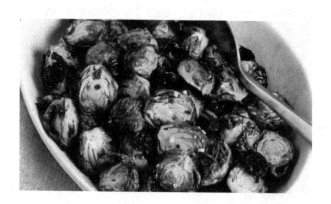

YIELDS: 4 SERVINGS | PREP TIME: 0 HOURS 10 MINS | TOTAL TIME: 0 HOURS 30 MINS

INGREDIENTS

- 1 lb. Brussels grows, managed and cut down the middle
- 1 tbsp. extra-virgin olive oil
- Genuine salt
- Newly ground dark pepper
- Squeeze squashed red pepper drops
- Juice of 1/2 lemon
- 1 tbsp. nectar
- 1 tbsp. red wine vinegar
- 2 tsp. Dijon mustard
- 1 clove garlic, minced

DIRECTIONS

1. In a medium bowl, add Brussels fledglings and oil and season with salt, pepper, and red pepper pieces. Throw around to cover Brussels grows well.

2. Add Brussels fledglings to container of air fryer, working in clumps depending on the situation, and cook at 380° for 18 minutes, halting and throwing Brussels in bin part of the way through.
3. In the interim, make dressing: In a little bowl, whisk together lemon juice, nectar, vinegar, mustard, and garlic. Season with salt and pepper.
4. Add cooked Brussels grows back to a medium blow away and pour dressing and throw to join.

3.   Antipasto Egg Rolls

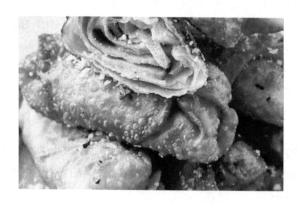

YIELDS: 12 | PREP TIME: 0 HOURS 10 MINS | TOTAL TIME: 0 HOURS 30 MINS

INGREDIENTS

- 12 egg move coverings
- 12 cuts provolone
- 12 cuts shop ham
- 36 cuts pepperoni
- 1 c. shredded mozzarella
- 1 c. cut pepperoncini
- Vegetable oil, for fricasseeing on burner
- 1/4 c. newly ground Parmesan
- Italian dressing, for serving

DIRECTIONS
FOR STOVETOP

1. Spot an egg move covering on a perfect surface in a precious stone shape place a cut of provolone in the middle. Top with one cut of ham, 3 cuts of pepperoni, and a huge spot of both mozzarella and pepperoncini. Overlay up base half and firmly crease in sides. Tenderly

move, at that point seal overlap several drops of water.
2. In a huge skillet over medium heat, heat oil (it should arrive at 1" up the side of container) until it pops and air pockets when a drop of water is added to the dish. Add egg rolls and fry until brilliant, 1 moment for each side; at that point move to a paper towel-lined plate.
3. Enhancement with Parmesan and parsley and serve quickly, with Italian dressing as an afterthought for plunging.

FOR AIR FRYER

1. Spot an egg move covering on a perfect surface in a precious stone shape place a cut of provolone in the middle. Top with one cut of ham, 3 cuts of pepperoni, and an enormous spot of both mozzarella and pepperoncini. Overlap up base half and firmly crease in sides. Tenderly move, at that point seal overlap several drops of water.
2. Working in bunches, cook egg moves at 390° until brilliant, around 12 minutes, flipping partially through.

4. Air Fryer Chicken Tenders

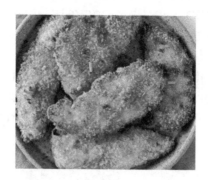

YIELDS: 4 SERVINGS | PREP TIME: 0 HOURS 15 MINS | TOTAL TIME: 1 HOUR 0 MINS

INGREDIENTS

FOR THE CHICKEN TENDERS

- 1/2 lb. chicken fingers
- Genuine salt
- Newly ground dark pepper
- 1/2 c. generally useful flour
- 2 1/2 c. panko bread scraps
- 2 huge eggs
- 1/4 c. buttermilk
- Cooking splash

FOR THE HONEY MUSTARD

- 1/3 c. mayonnaise
- 3 tbsp. nectar
- 2 tbsp. Dijon mustard
- 1/4 tsp. hot sauce (optional)
- Spot of genuine salt
- Newly ground dark pepper

DIRECTIONS

1. Season chicken strips on the two sides with salt and pepper. Spot flour and bread morsels in two separate shallow dishes. In a third bowl, whisk together eggs and buttermilk. Working each in turn, dunk chicken in flour, at that point egg blend, lastly in bread pieces, squeezing to cover.

2. Working in groups, place chicken fingers in crate of air fryer, being certain to not pack it. Splash the highest points of chicken with cooking shower and cook at 400° for 5 minutes. Flip chicken over; shower the tops with really cooking splash and cook 5 minutes more. Rehash with staying chicken strips.

3. Make sauce: In a little bowl, whisk together mayonnaise, nectar, Dijon, and hot sauce, if using. Season with a spot of salt and a couple of breaks of dark pepper.

4. Serve chicken fingers with nectar mustard.

5. Air Fryer Chicken Parmesan

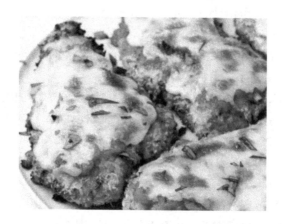

YIELDS: 4 SERVINGS | PREP TIME: 0 HOURS 10 MINS | TOTAL TIME: 0 HOURS 50 MINS

INGREDIENTS

- 2 huge boneless chicken breasts
- Genuine salt
- Newly ground dark pepper
- 1/3 c. generally useful flour
- 2 huge eggs
- 1 c. panko bread scraps
- 1/4 c. newly ground Parmesan
- 1 tsp. dried oregano
- 1/2 tsp. garlic powder
- 1/2 tsp. squashed red pepper pieces
- 1 c. marinara sauce
- 1 c. shredded mozzarella
- Newly chopped parsley, for embellish

DIRECTIONS

1. Cautiously butterfly chicken by slicing down the middle widthwise to make 4 slim bits of chicken. Season on the two sides with salt and pepper.
2. Get ready digging station: Place flour in a shallow bowl and season with a huge spot of salt and pepper. Spot eggs in a subsequent bowl and beat. In a third bowl, join bread scraps, Parmesan, oregano, garlic powder, and red pepper chips.
3. Working with each piece of a chicken in turn, coat in flour, at that point dunk in eggs, and lastly press into panko blend ensuring the two sides are covered well.
4. Working in clusters as important, place chicken in bushel of air fryer and cook at 400° for 5 minutes on each side. Top chicken with sauce and mozzarella and cook at 400° for 3 minutes more or until cheddar is melty and brilliant.
5. Enhance with parsley to serve.

6.   Cheesy Beef Empanadas

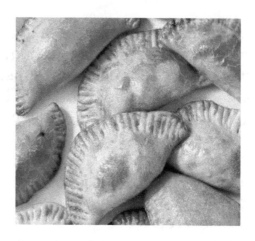

YIELDS: 15 PREP TIME: 0 HOURS 20 MINS TOTAL TIME: 2 HOURS 0 MINS

INGREDIENTS
FOR THE DOUGH

- 3 c. generally useful flour, in addition to additional for surface
- 1 tsp. legitimate salt
- 1 tsp. preparing powder
- 1/2 c. cold margarine, cut into 3D shapes
- 3/4 c. water
- 1 enormous egg

FOR THE BEEF FILLING

- 1 tbsp. extra-virgin olive oil
- 1 yellow onion, chopped
- 2 cloves garlic, minced
- 1 lb. ground meat
- 1 tbsp. tomato paste
- 1 tsp. oregano

- 1 tsp. cumin
- 1/2 tsp. paprika
- Legitimate salt
- Newly ground dark pepper
- 1/2 c. chopped tomatoes
- 1/2 c. chopped cured jalapeños
- 1/4 c. shredded Cheddar
- 1/4 c. Shredded Monterey Jack
- Egg wash, for brushing
- Newly chopped cilantro, for embellish
- Sharp cream, for serving

DIRECTIONS
MAKE DOUGH

1. In an enormous bowl, whisk together flour, salt, and preparing powder. Cut margarine into flour using your hands or a baked good shaper until pea-sized. Add water and egg and blend until a batter structures. Turn mixture out on a softly floured surface and work until smooth, around 5 minutes.
2. Enclose by saran wrap and refrigerate for at any rate 60 minutes.

FOR OVEN

1. Preheat oven to 400° and fix two huge heating sheets with material paper.
2. In an enormous skillet over medium heat, heat oil. Add onion and cook until delicate, around 5 minutes, at that point add garlic and cook until fragrant, brief more. Add ground hamburger and cook, separating meat with a wooden spoon, until not, at this point pink, 5 minutes. Channel fat.

3. Return skillet to medium heat, and mix tomato paste into meat. Add oregano, cumin, and paprika, and season with salt and pepper. Add tomatoes and jalapeños and cook until warmed through, around 3 minutes. Eliminate from heat and let cool marginally.
4. Spot mixture on a daintily floured surface and gap down the middle. Carry one half out to ¼" thick. Using a 4.5" round cutout, cut out adjusts. Rehash with residual batter. Reroll scraps once to remove more adjusts.
5. Gently dampen external edge of a mixture round with water and spot around 2 tablespoons filling in focus and top with cheddar and Monterey. Overlay mixture fifty-fifty over filling. Utilize a fork to pleat edges together. Rehash with outstanding filling and batter.
6. Spot empanadas on arranged heating sheets and brush with egg wash. Heat until brilliant and filling is warmed through, around 25 minutes.
7. Embellishment with cilantro and present with acrid cream.

FOR AIR FRYER

1. In a huge skillet over medium heat, heat oil. Add onion and cook until delicate, around 5 minutes, at that point add garlic and cook until fragrant, brief more. Add ground hamburger and cook, separating meat with a wooden spoon, until not, at this point pink, 5 minutes. Channel fat.

2. Return dish to medium heat, and mix tomato paste into hamburger. Add oregano, cumin, and paprika, and season with salt and pepper. Add tomatoes and jalapeños and cook until warmed through, around 3 minutes. Eliminate from heat and let cool somewhat.
3. Spot batter on a gently floured surface and gap into equal parts. Carry one half out to ¼" thick. Using a 4.5" round cutout, cut out adjusts. Rehash with residual mixture. Reroll scraps once to remove more adjusts.
4. Gently dampen external edge of a mixture round with water and spot around 2 tablespoons filling in focus and top with cheddar and Monterey. Crease batter down the middle over filling. Utilize a fork to crease edges together, at that point brush with egg wash. Rehash with residual filling and mixture.
5. Spot empanadas in a material lined Air Fryer crate, ensuring they don't contact, and cook in clumps at 400° for 10 minutes.
6. Enhance with cilantro and present with harsh cream.

7.   Bacon Avocado Fries

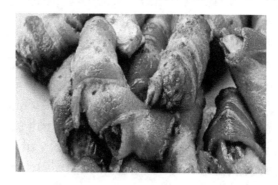

CAL/SERV: 120 | YIELDS: 24 | PREP TIME: 0 HOURS 5 MINS | COOK TIME: 0 HOURS 0 MINS | TOTAL TIME: 0 HOURS 5 MINS

INGREDIENTS
- 3 avocados
- 24 flimsy segments of bacon
- 1/4 c. farm dressing, for serving

DIRECTIONS
FOR OVEN
1. Preheat oven to 425º. Cut every avocado into 8 similarly estimated wedges. Envelop each wedge by bacon, cutting bacon if necessary. Spot on a preparing sheet, crease side down.
2. Heat until bacon is cooked through and firm, 12 to 15 minutes.
3. Present with farm dressing.

FOR AIR FRYER

1. Cut every avocado into 8 similarly measured wedges. Wrap each wedge with a segment of bacon, cutting bacon if necessary.
2. Working in clusters, orchestrate in air fryer bin in a solitary layer. Cook at 400° for 8 minutes until bacon is cooked through and firm.
3. Serve warm with farm.

8.   Homemade Cannoli

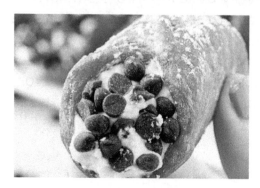

YIELDS: 20 | PREP TIME: 0 HOURS 10 MINS | TOTAL
TIME: 3 HOURS 0 MINS

INGREDIENTS
FOR THE FILLING:

- 1 (16-oz.) compartment ricotta
- 1/2 c. mascarpone cheddar
- 1/2 c. powdered sugar, partitioned
- 3/4 c. weighty cream
- 1 tsp. unadulterated vanilla concentrate
- 1 tsp. orange zing
- 1/4 tsp. genuine salt
- 1/2 c. small scale chocolate chips, for decorate

FOR THE SHELLS:

- 2 c. universally handy flour, in addition to additional for surface
- 1/4 c. granulated sugar
- 1 tsp. genuine salt
- 1/2 tsp. cinnamon
- 4 tbsp. cold spread, cut into 3D shapes
- 6 tbsp. white wine
- 1 huge egg
- 1 egg white, for brushing
- Vegetable oil, for fricasseeing

DIRECTIONS
MAKE FILLING:

1. Channel ricotta by putting it a fine lattice sifter set over a huge bowl. Give channel access cooler for in any event an hour and up to expedite.
2. In an enormous bowl using a hand blender, beat weighty cream and 1/4 cup powdered sugar until hardened pinnacles structure.
3. In another huge bowl, consolidate ricotta, mascarpone, staying 1/4 cup powdered sugar, vanilla, orange zing, and salt. Overlay in whipped cream. Refrigerate until prepared to fill cannoli, at any rate 60 minutes.

MAKE SHELLS:

1. In a huge bowl, whisk together flour, sugar, salt, and cinnamon. Cut spread into flour blend with your hands or cake shaper until pea-sized. Add wine and egg and blend until a batter structures. Massage a couple of times in bowl to help batter meet up. Pat into a level circle, at that point envelop by saran wrap and refrigerate at any rate 1 hour and up to expedite.
2. On a gently floured surface, partition mixture fifty-fifty. Carry one half out to ⅛" thick. Utilize a 4" circle cutout to remove batter. Rehash with residual mixture. Re-move scraps to cut a couple of additional circles.
3. Fold batter over cannoli shape and brush egg whites where the mixture will meet to seal together.

FOR FRYING:

1. In an enormous pot over medium heat, heat around 2" of oil to 360°. Working in clumps, add cannoli molds to oil and broil, turning infrequently, until brilliant, around 4 minutes. Eliminate from oil and spot on a paper towel-lined plate. Let cool marginally.
2. At the point when sufficiently cool to deal with or using a kitchen towel to hold, delicately bend shells off of molds to eliminate.
3. Spot filling in a cake pack fitted with an open star tip. Line filling into shells, at that point plunge closes in small scale chocolate chips.

FOR AIR FRYER:

1. Working in clusters, place molds in bin of air fryer and cook at 350° for 12 minutes, or until brilliant.
2. At the point when sufficiently cool to deal with or using a kitchen towel to hold, delicately eliminate curve shells off of molds.
3. Spot filling in a baked good sack fitted with an open star tip. Line filling into shells, at that point plunge closes in smaller than expected chocolate chips.

9.   Twice Baked Potatoes

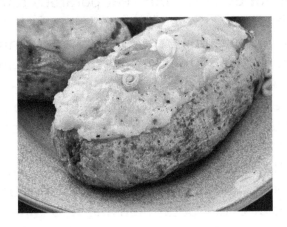

YIELDS: 6 SERVINGS | PREP TIME: 0 HOURS 10
MINS | TOTAL TIME: 2 HOURS 0 MINS

INGREDIENTS

- 6 huge reddish brown potatoes, thoroughly cleaned
- 1 tbsp. extra-virgin olive oil
- Legitimate salt
- 1/2 c. (1 stick) margarine, relaxed
- 1/2 c. milk
- 1/2 c. sharp cream
- 1/2 c. shredded Cheddar, separated
- 2 green onions, daintily cut, in addition to additional for decorate
- Newly ground dark pepper

DIRECTIONS
FOR OVEN

1. Preheat oven to 400°. Pat potatoes totally dry with paper towels. Jab potatoes done with a fork, at that point rub with oil and sprinkle with salt. Spot potatoes straightforwardly on oven racks and prepare until potatoes are penetrated effectively with a fork, around 60 minutes. Spot on a huge heating sheet and let cool until adequately cool to deal with.

2. Cutting longwise cut a slim layer off the highest point of every potato. Scoop back to front of every potato leaving a ½" line. Spot internal parts in an enormous bowl. Keep the potato tops and dish them on the plate as a tidbit!

3. To bowl with potatoes, add margarine, milk, and sharp cream and crush until spread is softened in and potatoes are for the most part smooth, yet for certain pieces. Add 1 cup of cheddar and green onions and mix until fused. Season with salt and pepper.

4. Fill heated potatoes with potato blend and spot on a huge preparing sheet. Top with remaining ½ cup of cheddar. Heat until cheddar is melty and outside is fresh, 15 minutes.

5. Trimming with more green onions prior to serving.

FOR AIR FRYER

1. Pat potatoes totally dry with paper towels. Jab potatoes done with a fork, at that point rub with oil and sprinkle with salt. Working in groups, place potatoes in crate of air fryer and cook on 400° for 40 minutes. Spot on a huge preparing sheet and let cool until sufficiently cool to deal with.

2. Cutting longwise cut a dainty layer off the highest point of every potato. Scoop back to front of every potato leaving a ½" line. Spot inner parts in an enormous bowl. Keep the potato tops and dish them on the plate as a tidbit!

3. To bowl with potatoes, add spread, milk, and harsh cream and crush until margarine is dissolved in and potatoes are for the most part smooth, however for certain pieces. Add 1 cup of cheddar and green onions and mix until joined. Season with salt and pepper.

4. Fill heated potatoes with potato blend and spot back in bushel of air fryer. Top with remaining ½ cup of cheddar. Cook at 400° until cheddar is melty and outside is fresh, 5 minutes.

5. Trim with more green onions prior to serving.

10. Spicy Chicken Taquitos

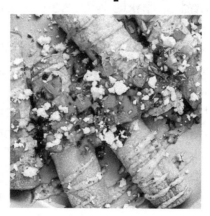

YIELDS: 12 | PREP TIME: 0 HOURS 15 MINS | TOTAL TIME: 0 HOURS 45 MINS

INGREDIENTS
FOR TAQUITOS

- Cooking splash
- 3 c. shredded cooked chicken
- 1 (8-oz.) block cream cheddar, mollified
- 1 chipotle in adobo sauce, chopped, in addition to 1 tbsp. sauce
- 1 tsp. cumin
- 1 tsp. stew powder
- Legitimate salt
- Newly ground dark pepper
- 12 little corn tortillas
- 1/2 c. shredded cheddar
- 1/2 c. shredded Pepper Jack
- Pico de Gallo, for serving
- Disintegrated queso fresco, for serving

FOR AVOCADO CREAM SAUCE
- 1 huge avocado, pitted
- 1/2 c. sharp cream
- 1/4 c. stuffed cilantro leaves
- 1 clove garlic
- Juice of lime
- Legitimate salt
- Newly ground dark pepper

DIRECTIONS
FOR OVEN:
1. Preheat oven to 425° and oil a huge preparing sheet with cooking splash. In a huge bowl, join chicken, cream cheddar, chipotle and sauce, cumin, and stew powder. Season with salt and pepper.
2. Spot tortillas on a microwave safe plate and cover with a moist paper towel. Microwave 30 seconds, or until warm and more flexible.
3. Spread about ¼ cup of filling toward one side of tortilla, at that point sprinkle a tad bit of cheddar and pepper jack close to filling. Move up firmly and place crease side down on preparing sheet. Rehash with outstanding filling and cheddar.
4. Heat until fresh and brilliant, 15 to 20 minutes.
5. Present with avocado cream sauce, Pico de Gallo, and queso fresco

FOR AIR FRYER:
1. In an enormous bowl, join chicken, cream cheddar, chipotle and sauce, cumin, and stew powder. Season with salt and pepper.

2. Spot tortillas on a microwave safe plate and cover with a clammy paper towel. Microwave 30 seconds, or until warm and more malleable.
3. Spread about ¼ cup of filling toward one side of tortilla, at that point sprinkle a tad bit of cheddar and pepper jack close to filling. Move up firmly. Rehash with residual filling and cheddar.
4. Spot in crate of air fryer, crease side down, and cook at 400° for 7 minutes.
5. Present with avocado cream sauce, Pico de Gallo, and queso fresco.

FOR AVOCADO CREAM SAUCE:
1. In a food processor, mix together avocado, acrid cream, cilantro, garlic, and lime juice. Season with salt and pepper. Fill a bowl and press plastic wrap straightforwardly over surface and refrigerate until prepared to utilize.

11. Air Fryer Pizza

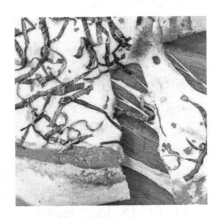

YIELDS: 2 SERVINGS | PREP TIME: 0 HOURS 10 MINS | TOTAL TIME: 0 HOURS 10 MINS

INGREDIENTS

- 2 (8-oz.) bundles pizza mixture
- 1 tbsp. additional virgin olive oil, partitioned
- 1/3 c. squashed tomatoes
- 1 clove garlic, minced
- 1/2 tsp. oregano
- Genuine salt
- Newly ground dark pepper
- 1/2 (8-oz.) mozzarella ball, cut into ¼" cuts
- Basil leaves, for serving

DIRECTIONS

1. On a clean, floured surface, delicately level bundle of batter with your hands until around 8" in breadth (or generally more modest than your air fryer bin). Rehash with second batter ball. Brush both with olive oil and move one, oil side up, into the container of your air fryer.

2. In a medium bowl, mix to join squashed tomatoes, garlic, and oregano, and season with salt and pepper. Spoon half tomato blend onto the focal point of carried out pizza batter, at that point spread into an even layer, leaving ½" external outside uncovered.

3. Add a large portion of the mozzarella cuts to pizza. Air fry on 400° for 10 to 12 minutes, or until outside is brilliant and cheddar is dissolved.

4. Eliminate first pizza from air fryer container using 2 pairs of utensils, and enhancement with basil leaves. Collect and cook second pizza, trimming, and serve

12. Air Fryer Doughnuts

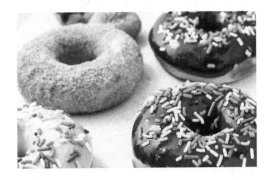

YIELDS: 6 | PREP TIME: 0 HOURS 10 MINS | TOTAL TIME: 2 HOURS 40 MINS

INGREDIENTS
FOR THE DONUTS
- Cooking shower
- 1/2 c. milk
- 1/4 c. furthermore 1 tsp. granulated sugar, isolated
- 1 (0.25-oz.) parcel or 2 1/4 tsp. dynamic dry yeast
- 2 c. universally handy flour
- 1/2 tsp. fit salt
- 4 tbsp. margarine, softened
- 1 enormous egg
- 1 tsp. unadulterated vanilla concentrate

FOR THE VANILLA GLAZE
- 1 c. powdered sugar
- 2 oz. milk
- 1/2 tsp. unadulterated vanilla concentrate

FOR THE CHOCOLATE GLAZE
- 3/4 c. powdered sugar
- 1/4 c. unsweetened cocoa powder

- 3 tbsp. milk
- FOR THE CINNAMON SUGAR
- 1/2 c. granulated sugar
- 2 tbsp. ground cinnamon
- 2 tbsp. softened margarine

DIRECTIONS
MAKE THE DOUGHNUTS
1. Oil a huge bowl with cooking shower. In a little, microwave-safe bowl or glass estimating cup, add milk. Microwave until tepid, 40 seconds. Add a teaspoon of sugar and mix to break up, at that point sprinkle over yeast and let sit until foamy, around 8 minutes.
2. In a medium bowl, whisk together flour and salt. In an enormous bowl, whisk together excess ¼ cup sugar, spread, egg, and vanilla. Pour in yeast blend, blend to consolidate, at that point include dry ingredients, mixing with a wooden spoon until a shaggy mixture structures.
3. Move to a softly floured surface and manipulate until flexible and just somewhat crude, adding more flour a teaspoon at an at once, around 5 minutes. Structure into a ball at that point place mixture in oiled bowl and cover with a perfect drying towel. Allow batter to ascend in a warm spot until multiplied in size, around 60 minutes.

4. Line a huge heating sheet with material paper and softly oil with cooking shower. Punch down batter, at that point turn onto a softly floured work surface and carry out into a ½" thick square shape.

5. Using a donut shaper or 3" and 1" roll cutters, finish off your doughnuts. Massage any pieces together and finish off more doughnuts or openings. Spot doughnuts and openings onto preparing sheets, cover with kitchen towel, and let rise once more, 40 minutes to 1 hour more.

6. Oil container of air fryer with cooking splash and add 2 doughnuts and 2 donut openings all at once, ensuring doughnuts don't contact. Cook at 375° for 6 minutes, until profoundly brilliant. Spot on cooling rack and rehash with outstanding mixture.

7. Dunk doughnuts in glaze (see beneath) or adhere to guidelines for cinnamon sugar. Get back to cooling rack and let set for 5 minutes prior to serving.

MAKE THE VANILLA GLAZE:
1. In a medium bowl whisk together powdered sugar, milk, and vanilla until smooth.

MAKE THE CHOCOLATE GLAZE:
1. In a medium bowl whisk together powdered sugar, cocoa powder, and milk.

MAKE THE CINNAMON SUGAR
1. In an enormous shallow bowl, whisk together cinnamon and sugar. Brush doughnuts with softened margarine and throw in cinnamon sugar.

13. Brussels Sprout Chips

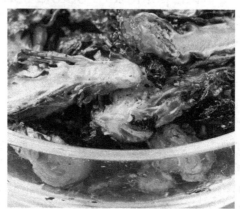

YIELDS: 2 - 3 SERVINGS | PREP TIME: 0 HOURS 5
MINS | TOTAL TIME: 0 HOURS 25 MINS

INGREDIENTS
- 1/2 lb. Brussels sprouts, meagerly cut
- 1 tbsp. extra-virgin olive oil
- 2 tbsp. newly ground Parmesan, in addition to additional for decorate
- 1 tsp. garlic powder
- Fit salt
- Newly ground dark pepper
- Caesar dressing, for plunging

DIRECTIONS
FOR OVEN
1. Preheat oven to 400°. In an enormous bowl, throw Brussels sprouts with oil, Parmesan, and garlic powder and season with salt and pepper. Spread in an even layer on a medium heating sheet.
2. Prepare 10 minutes, throw, and heat 8 to 10 minutes more, until fresh and brilliant.

Enhancement with more Parmesan and present with Caesar dressing for plunging.

FOR AIR FRYER

1. In a huge bowl, throw Brussels sprouts with oil, Parmesan, and garlic powder and season with salt and pepper. Mastermind in an even layer in air fryer.
2. Prepare at 350° for 8 minutes, throw, and heat 8 minutes more, until fresh and brilliant.
3. Embellish with more Parmesan and present with Caesar dressing for plunging.

14. Air Fryer Blooming Onion

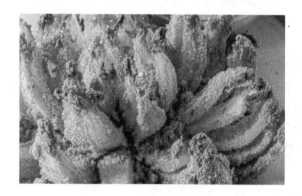

YIELDS: 4 SERVINGS | PREP TIME: 0 HOURS
15 MINS | TOTAL TIME: 0 HOURS 45 MINS

INGREDIENTS
FOR THE ONION

- 1 enormous yellow onion
- 3 enormous eggs
- 1 c. breadcrumbs
- 2 tsp. paprika
- 1 tsp. garlic powder
- 1 tsp. onion powder
- 1 tsp. genuine salt
- 3 tbsp. extra-virgin olive oil

FOR THE SAUCE

- 2/3 c. mayonnaise
- 2 tbsp. ketchup
- 1 tsp. horseradish
- 1/2 tsp. paprika
- 1/2 tsp. garlic powder
- 1/4 tsp. dried oregano

- Genuine salt

DIRECTIONS

1. Cut off onion stem and set onion on level side. Cut an inch starting from the root, into 12 to 16 segments, being mindful so as not to carve entirely through. Flip over and delicately pull out areas of onion to isolate petals.
2. In a shallow bowl, whisk together eggs and 1 tablespoon water. In another shallow bowl, whisk together breadcrumbs and flavors. Plunge onion into egg wash; at that point dig in breadcrumb blend, using a spoon to completely cover. Sprinkle onion with oil.
3. Spot in container of air fryer and cook at 375° until onion is delicate entirely through, 20 to 25 minutes. Shower with more oil as wanted.
4. In the interim make sauce: In a medium bowl, whisk together mayonnaise, ketchup, horseradish, paprika, garlic powder, and dried oregano. Season with salt.
5. Serve onion with sauce, for plunging.

15. Best-Ever Mozzarella Sticks

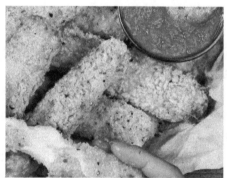

YIELDS: 6 | PREP TIME: 0 HOURS 5 MINS | TOTAL TIME: 2 HOURS 25 MINS

INGREDIENTS

- 6 mozzarella sticks
- 1 c. panko bread pieces
- Legitimate salt
- Newly broke dark pepper
- 2 huge eggs, very much beaten
- 3 tbsp. generally useful flour
- Warm marinara, for serving

DIRECTIONS
FOR OVEN

1. Freeze mozzarella sticks until frozen strong, in any event 2 hours.
2. At the point when prepared to bread, preheat oven to 400° and fix a little heating sheet with material paper. Set up a breading station: Place panko, eggs, and flour in 3 separate shallow dishes. Season panko liberally with salt and pepper.
3. Coat frozen mozzarella sticks in flour, at that point plunge in egg, at that point panko, back

in the egg, at that point back in the panko. Mastermind on a heating sheet.
4. Prepare for 8 to 10 minutes, observing cautiously so the cheddar doesn't overflow.
5. Present with warm marinara sauce for plunging.

FOR AIR FRYER
1. Freeze mozzarella sticks until frozen strong, in any event 2 hours.
2. Following 3 hours, set up a breading station: Place panko, eggs, and flour in 3 separate shallow dishes. Season panko liberally with salt and pepper.
3. Coat frozen mozzarella sticks in flour, at that point dunk in egg, at that point panko, back in the egg, at that point back in the panko.
4. Orchestrate frozen breaded mozzarella sticks in an even layer in the bushel of your air fryer. Cook on 400° for 6 minutes, or until brilliant and fresh outwardly and melty in the middle.
5. Present with warm marinara sauce for plunging.

16. Air Fryer Spicy Chicken Thighs

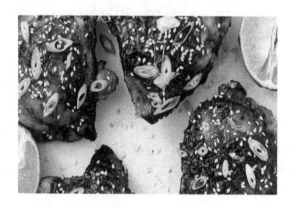

YIELDS: 4 SERVINGS | PREP TIME: 0 HOURS 10 MINS | TOTAL TIME: 1 HOUR 20 MINS

INGREDIENTS

- 1/3 c. low-sodium soy sauce
- 1/4 c. extra-virgin olive oil
- 2 tbsp. nectar
- 2 tbsp. bean stew garlic sauce
- Juice of 1 lime
- 2 cloves garlic, minced
- 2 tsp. newly ground ginger
- 4 bone-in, skin-on chicken thighs (around 2 lb.)
- Meagerly cut green onions, for embellish
- Toasted sesame seeds, for decorate

DIRECTIONS

1. In an enormous bowl, consolidate soy sauce, oil, nectar, stew garlic sauce, lime juice, garlic, and ginger. Save ½ cup of marinade. Add chicken thighs to bowl and throw to cover. Cover and refrigerate for in any event 30 minutes.
2. Eliminate 2 thighs from marinade and spot in crate of air fryer. Cook at 400° until thighs are cooked through to an inner temperature of 165°, 15 to 20 minutes. Move thighs to a plate and tent with foil. Rehash with outstanding thighs.
3. In the interim, in a little pot over medium heat, heat held marinade to the point of boiling. Lessen heat and stew until sauce thickens marginally, 4 to 5 minutes.
4. Brush sauce over thighs and topping with green onions and sesame seeds prior to serving.

17. Air fryer Apple Chips

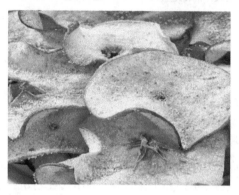

INGREDIENTS
- 2 apples, daintily cut
- 2 tsp. granulated sugar
- 1/2 tsp. cinnamon

DIRECTIONS
FOR OVEN
1. Preheat oven to 200°. In a huge bowl, throw apples with sugar and cinnamon.
2. Spot a metal rack inside a rimmed heating sheet. Lay apples cuts on top of rack, separating them so no apples cover.
3. Prepare for 2 to 3 hours, flipping apples partially through, until apples dried out yet flexible. (Apples will keep on crisping while at the same time cooling.)

FOR AIR FRYER
1. In a huge bowl throw apples with cinnamon and sugar. Working in groups, place apples in a solitary layer in bushel of air fryer (some cover is alright).
2. Prepare at 350° for around 12 minutes, flipping at regular intervals.

18. Air Fryer Cinnamon Rolls

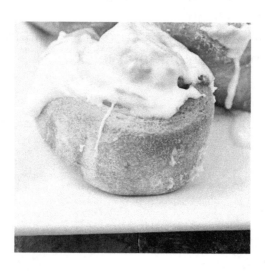

YIELDS: 6 | PREP TIME: 0 HOURS 5 MINS | TOTAL
TIME: 0 HOURS 30 MINS

INGREDIENTS
FOR THE ROLLS

- 2 tbsp. dissolved spread, in addition to additional for brushing
- 1/3 c. stuffed brown sugar
- 1/2 tsp. ground cinnamon
- Legitimate salt
- Generally useful flour, for surface
- 1 (8-oz.) tube refrigerated Crescent rolls

FOR THE GLAZE
- 2 oz. cream cheddar, mellowed
- 1/2 c. powdered sugar
- 1 tbsp. entire milk, in addition to more if necessary

DIRECTIONS
1. Make moves: Line lower part of air fryer with material paper and brush with margarine. In a medium bowl, consolidate spread, brown sugar, cinnamon, and an enormous spot of salt until smooth and cushioned.
2. On a daintily floured surface, carry out bow abounds in one piece. Squeeze creases together and overlap down the middle. Fold into a 9"- x-7" square shape. Spread margarine blend over batter, leaving 1/4-inch line. Beginning at a long edge, move up batter like a jam move, at that point cut transversely into 6 pieces.
3. Organize pieces in arranged air fryer, cut-side up, separated uniformly.
4. Set air fryer to 350°, and cook until brilliant and cooked through, around 10 minutes.
5. Make the coating: In a medium bowl, Whisk cream cheddar, powdered sugar, and milk together. Add more milk by the teaspoonful, if vital, to thin coating.
6. Spread coating over warm cinnamon rolls and serve.

19. Air Fryer Fried Chicken

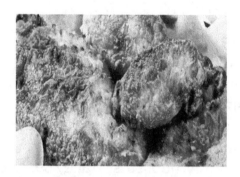

YIELDS: 3 SERVINGS | PREP TIME: 0 HOURS 10 MINS | TOTAL TIME: 2 HOURS 10 MINS

INGREDIENTS

- 2 lb. bone-in skin-on chicken pieces (blend of cuts)
- 2 c. buttermilk
- 1/2 c. hot sauce
- 3 tsp. fit salt, partitioned
- 2 c. universally handy flour
- 1 tsp. garlic powder
- 1 tsp. onion powder
- 1/2 tsp. oregano
- 1/2 tsp. newly ground dark pepper
- 1/4 tsp. cayenne pepper

DIRECTIONS

1. Cut back chicken of abundance excess and spot in an enormous bowl. In a medium bowl, join buttermilk, hot sauce, and 2 teaspoons salt.

2. Pour combination over chicken, ensuring all pieces are covered. Cover and refrigerate for in any event 1 hour and up to expedite.
3. In a shallow bowl or pie dish, consolidate flour, staying 1 teaspoon salt, and flavors. Working with each in turn, eliminates chicken from buttermilk, shaking off overabundance buttermilk. Spot in flour blend, going to cover.
4. Spot covered chicken in bushel of air fryer, working in bunches as important to not pack the bin. Cook at 400° until chicken is brilliant and inward temperature arrives at 165°, 20 to 25 minutes, flipping partially through.
5. Rehash with staying chicken.

20. Air-Fryer Ground Beef Wellington

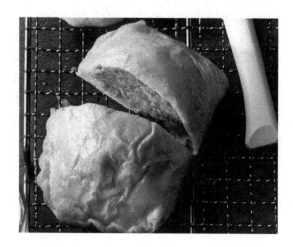

Prep: 30 min. Cook: 20 min. | makes: 2 servings

Ingredients

- 1 tablespoon spread
- 1/2 cup chopped new mushrooms
- 2 teaspoons generally useful flour
- 1/4 teaspoon pepper, separated
- 1/2 cup creamer cream
- 1 huge egg yolk
- 2 tablespoons finely chopped onion
- 1/4 teaspoon salt
- 1/2 pound ground meat
- 1 cylinder (4 ounces) refrigerated sickle rolls
- 1 huge egg, daintily beaten, optional
- 1 teaspoon dried parsley chips

Directions

1. Preheat air fryer to 300°. In a pot, heat margarine over medium-high heat. Add mushrooms; cook and mix until delicate, 5-6 minutes. Mix in flour and 1/8 teaspoon pepper until mixed. Progressively add cream. Heat to the point of boiling; cook and mix for 2 minutes or until thickened. Eliminate from the heat and put in a safe spot.
2. In a bowl, join egg yolk, onion, 2 tablespoons mushroom sauce, salt and staying 1/8 teaspoon pepper. Disintegrate meat over blend and blend well. Shape into 2 portions. Unroll sickle batter and separate into 2 square shapes; press holes to seal. Spot meat portion on every square shape. Unite edges and squeeze to seal. Whenever wanted, brush with beaten egg.
3. Spot Wellingtons in a solitary layer on lubed plate in air-fryer bin. Cook until brilliant brown and a thermometer embedded into meat portion peruses 160°, 18-22 minutes.
4. In the meantime, warm leftover sauce over low heat; mix in parsley. Serve sauce with Wellingtons.

21. Air-Fryer Caribbean Wontons

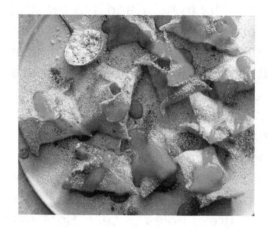

Total Time | Prep: 30 min. Cook: 10 min. /batch
Makes | 2 dozen (1-1/4 cups sauce)

Ingredients

- 4 ounces cream cheddar, relaxed
- 1/4 cup improved shredded coconut
- 1/4 cup pounded ready banana
- 2 tablespoons chopped pecans
- 2 tablespoons canned squashed pineapple
- 1 cup marshmallow creme
- 24 wonton coverings
- Cooking shower

SAUCE:

- 1 pound new strawberries, hulled
- 1/4 cup sugar
- 1 teaspoon cornstarch
- Confectioners' sugar and ground cinnamon

Directions

1. Preheat air fryer to 350°. In a little bowl, beat cream cheddar until smooth. Mix in coconut, banana, pecans and pineapple. Overlap in marshmallow crème.

2. Position a wonton covering with 1 highlights you. Continue to remain coverings covered with a sodden paper towel until prepared to utilize. Spot 2 teaspoons filling in the focal point of covering. Soak edges with water; crease inverse corners together over filling and press to seal. Rehash with residual coverings and filling.

3. In groups, orchestrate wontons in a solitary layer on lubed plate in air-fryer bin; spritz with cooking shower. Cook until brilliant brown and fresh, 10-12 minutes.

4. In the mean time, place strawberries in a food processor; cover and cycle until pureed. In a little pan, join sugar and cornstarch. Mix in pureed strawberries. Heat to the point of boiling; cook and mix until thickened, 2 minutes. Whenever wanted, strain blend, saving sauce; dispose of seeds. Sprinkle wontons with confectioners' sugar and cinnamon. Present with sauce.

22. Air-Fryer Wasabi Crab Cakes

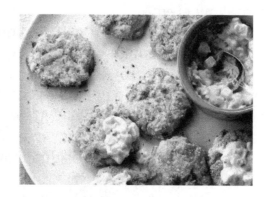

Total Time | Prep: 20 min. Cook: 10 min. /batch
Makes: 2 dozen (1/2 cup sauce)

Ingredients
- 1 medium sweet red pepper, finely chopped
- 1 celery rib, finely chopped
- 3 green onions, finely chopped
- 2 huge egg whites
- 3 tablespoons decreased fat mayonnaise
- 1/4 teaspoon arranged wasabi
- 1/4 teaspoon salt
- 1/3 cup in addition to 1/2 cup dry bread morsels, separated
- 1-1/2 cups irregularity crabmeat, depleted
- Cooking splash

SAUCE:
- 1 celery rib, chopped
- 1/3 cup decreased fat mayonnaise
- 1 green onion, chopped
- 1 tablespoon sweet pickle relish
- 1/2 teaspoon arranged wasabi

- 1/4 teaspoon celery salt

Directions
1. Preheat air fryer to 375°. Consolidate initial 7 ingredients; add 1/3 cup bread morsels. Tenderly crease in crab.
2. Spot remaining bread pieces in a shallow bowl. Drop piling tablespoons of crab blend into morsels. Tenderly coat and shape into 3/4-in. - thick patties. In groups, place crab cakes in a solitary layer on lubed plate in air-fryer crate. Spritz crab cakes with cooking shower. Cook until brilliant brown, 8-12 minutes, cautiously turning partially through cooking and spritzing with extra cooking shower.
3. In the interim, place sauce ingredients in food processor; beat 2 or multiple times to mix or until wanted consistency are reached. Serve crab cakes promptly with plunging sauce.

23. Air-Fryer Apple Fritters

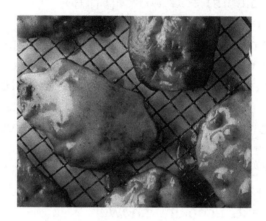

Prep: 10 min. Cook: 8 min. /batch | makes: 15 servings

Ingredients
Cooking splash

- 1-1/2 cups universally handy flour
- 1/4 cup sugar
- 2 teaspoons heating powder
- 1-1/2 teaspoons ground cinnamon
- 1/2 teaspoon salt
- 2/3 cup 2% milk
- 2 huge eggs, room temperature
- 1 tablespoon lemon juice
- 1-1/2 teaspoons vanilla concentrate, separated
- 2 medium Honey crisp apples, stripped and chopped
- 1/4 cup spread
- 1 cup confectioners' sugar
- 1 tablespoon 2% milk

Directions

1. Line air-fryer crate with material (slice to fit); spritz with cooking shower. Preheat air fryer to 410&deg.
2. In an enormous bowl, consolidate flour, sugar, heating powder, cinnamon and salt. Add milk, eggs, lemon juice and 1 teaspoon vanilla concentrate; mix just until saturated. Crease in apples.
3. In groups, drop mixture by 1/4 cupful's 2-in. separated onto air-fryer bin. Spritz with cooking splash. Cook until brilliant brown, 5-6 minutes. Turn squanders; keep on airing fry until brilliant brown, 1-2 minutes.
4. Dissolve margarine in little pot over medium-high heat. Cautiously cook until margarine begins to brown and froth, 5 minutes. Eliminate from heat; cool marginally. Add confectioners' sugar, 1 tablespoon milk and staying 1/2 teaspoon vanilla concentrate to browned margarine; rush until smooth. Sprinkle over squanders prior to serving.

24. Air-Fryer Carrot Coffee Cake

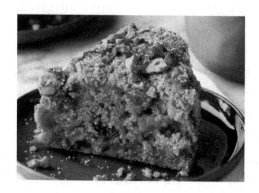

Prep: 15 min. Bake: 35 min. | Makes: 6 servings

Ingredients

- 1 enormous egg, gently beaten, room temperature
- 1/2 cup buttermilk
- 1/3 cup sugar in addition to 2 tablespoons sugar, partitioned
- 3 tablespoons canola oil
- 2 tablespoons dim brown sugar
- 1 teaspoon ground orange zing
- 1 teaspoon vanilla concentrate
- 2/3 cup universally handy flour
- 1/3 cup white entire wheat flour
- 1 teaspoon heating powder
- 2 teaspoons pumpkin pie zest, partitioned
- 1/4 teaspoon preparing pop
- 1/4 teaspoon salt
- 1 cup shredded carrots
- 1/4 cup dried cranberries
- 1/3 cup chopped pecans, toasted

Directions

1. Preheat air fryer to 350° Oil and flour a 6-in. round preparing dish. In a huge bowl, whisk egg, buttermilk, 1/3 cup sugar, oil, brown sugar, orange zing and vanilla. In another bowl, whisk flours, preparing powder, 1 teaspoon pumpkin pie zest, heating pop and salt. Continuously beat into egg blend. Overlap in carrots and dried cranberries. Fill arranged dish.
2. In a little bowl, consolidate pecans, staying 2 tablespoons sugar and staying 1 teaspoon pumpkin zest. Sprinkle equally over player. Delicately place skillet in the crate of a huge air fryer.
3. Cook until a toothpick embedded in focus confesses all, 35-40 minutes. Cover firmly with foil if top gets excessively dim. Cool in container on a wire rack for 10 minutes prior to eliminating from dish. Serve warm.

25. Air-Fryer Greek Breadsticks

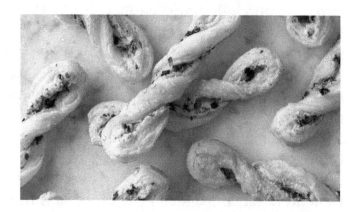

Prep: 20 min. Cook: 15 min. /batch | makes: 32 breadsticks

Ingredients

- 1/4 cup marinated quartered artichoke hearts, depleted
- 2 tablespoons pitted Greek olives
- 1 bundle (17.3 ounces) frozen puff cake, defrosted
- 1 container (6-1/2 ounces) spreadable spinach and artichoke cream cheddar
- 2 tablespoons ground Parmesan cheddar
- 1 huge egg
- 1 tablespoon water
- 2 teaspoons sesame seeds
- Refrigerated tzatziki sauce, optional

Directions

1. Preheat air fryer to 325°. Spot artichokes and olives in a food processor; cover and heartbeat until finely chopped. Unfurl 1 cake sheet on a daintily floured surface; spread a large portion of the cream cheddar over portion of cake. Top with a large portion of the artichoke combination. Sprinkle with a large portion of the Parmesan cheddar. Overlay plain half over filling; press delicately to seal.

2. Rehash with residual baked good, cream cheddar, artichoke combination and Parmesan cheddar. Whisk egg and water; brush over tops. Sprinkle with sesame seeds. Cut every square shape into sixteen 3/4-in. - wide strips. Bend strips a few times.

3. In groups, organize bread sticks in a solitary layer on lubed plate in air-fryer bushel. Cook until brilliant brown, 12-15 minutes. Serve warm with tzatziki sauce whenever wanted.

26. Cheesy Breakfast Egg Rolls

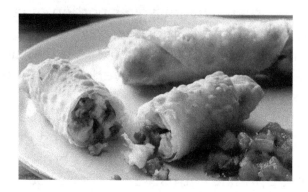

Prep: 30 min. Cook: 10 min. /batch | makes: 12 servings

Ingredients

- 1/2 pound mass pork frankfurter
- 1/2 cup shredded sharp cheddar
- 1/2 cup shredded Monterey Jack cheddar
- 1 tablespoon chopped green onions
- 4 enormous eggs
- 1 tablespoon 2% milk
- 1/4 teaspoon salt
- 1/8 teaspoon pepper
- 1 tablespoon margarine
- 12 egg move coverings
- Cooking shower
- Maple syrup or salsa, optional

Directions

1. In a little nonstick skillet, cook hotdog over medium heat until not, at this point pink, 4-6 minutes, breaking into disintegrates; channel. Mix in cheeses and green onions; put in a safe spot. Wipe skillet clean.
2. In a little bowl, whisk eggs, milk, salt and pepper until mixed. In a similar skillet, heat margarine over medium heat. Pour in egg combination; cook and mix until eggs are thickened and no fluid egg remains. Mix in wiener blend.
3. Preheat air fryer to 400°. With 1 corner of an egg move covering confronting you, place 1/4 cup filling just beneath focal point of covering. (Cover remaining coverings with a clammy paper towel until prepared to utilize.) Fold base corner over filling; soak remaining covering edges with water. Overlay side corners toward focus over filling. Move egg move up firmly, squeezing at tip to seal. Rehash.
4. In clumps, organize egg abounds in a solitary layer on lubed plate in air-fryer bin; spritz with cooking splash. Cook until softly browned, 3-4 minutes. Turn; spritz with cooking shower. Cook until brilliant brown and fresh, 3-4 minutes longer. Whenever wanted, present with maple syrup or salsa.

27. Air-Fryer Nacho Hot Dogs

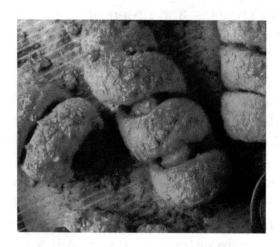

Prep: 20 min. Cook: 15 min. | makes: 6 servings

Ingredients

- 6 franks
- 3 cheddar sticks, divided the long way
- 1-1/4 cups self-rising flour
- 1 cup plain Greek yogurt
- 1/4 cup salsa
- 1/4 teaspoon bean stew powder
- 3 tablespoons chopped cultivated jalapeno pepper
- 1 cup squashed nacho-enhanced tortilla chips, separated
- Guacamole and harsh cream, optional

Directions

1. Cut a cut down the length of each frank without slicing through; embed a split cheddar stick into the cut. Put in a safe spot.

2. Preheat air fryer to 350°. In a huge bowl, mix together flour, yogurt, salsa, stew powder, jalapenos and ¼ cup squashed tortilla chips to shape a delicate batter. Spot mixture on a delicately floured surface; partition into sixths. Fold mixture into 15-inch long strips; fold one strip over cheddar stuffed sausage. Rehash with residual mixture and franks. Splash canines with cooking shower and tenderly move in leftover squashed chips. Splash air fryer container with cooking shower, and spot canines in bushel without contacting, leaving space to extend.

3. In groups, cook until mixture is somewhat browned and cheddar begins to soften, 8-10 minutes. Whenever wanted, present with extra salsa, sharp cream and guacamole.

28. Air-Fryer General Tso's Cauliflower

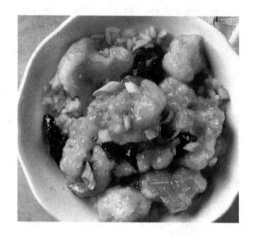

Prep: 25 min. Cook: 20 min. | Makes: 4 servings

Ingredients
- 1/2 cup all-purpose flour
- 1/2 cup cornstarch
- 1 teaspoon salt
- 1 teaspoon heating powder
- 3/4 cup club pop
- 1 medium head cauliflower, cut into 1-inch florets (around 6 cups)

SAUCE:
- 1/4 cup squeezed orange
- 3 tablespoons sugar
- 3 tablespoons soy sauce
- 3 tablespoons vegetable stock
- 2 tablespoons rice vinegar
- 2 teaspoons sesame oil
- 2 teaspoons cornstarch

- 2 tablespoons canola oil
- 2 to 6 dried pasilla or other hot chilies, chopped
- 3 green onions, white part minced, green part daintily cut
- 3 garlic cloves, minced
- 1 teaspoon ground new gingerroot
- 1/2 teaspoon ground orange zing
- 4 cups hot cooked rice

Directions

1. Preheat air fryer to 400°. Join flour, cornstarch, salt and heating powder. Mix in club soft drink just until mixed (player will be slim). Throw florets in hitter; move to a wire rack set over a heating sheet. Let stand 5 minutes. In groups, place cauliflower on lubed plate in air-fryer bushel. Cook until brilliant brown and delicate, 10-12 minutes.
2. Then, whisk together initial 6 sauce ingredients; rush in cornstarch until smooth.
3. In an enormous pan, heat canola oil over medium-high heat. Add chilies; cook and mix until fragrant, 1-2 minutes. Add white piece of onions, garlic, ginger and orange zing; cook until fragrant, around 1 moment. Mix squeezed orange blend; add to pot. Heat to the point of boiling; cook and mix until thickened, 2-4 minutes.
4. Add cauliflower to sauce; throw to cover. Present with rice; sprinkle with daintily cut green onions.

29. Air-Fryer Pork Schnitzel

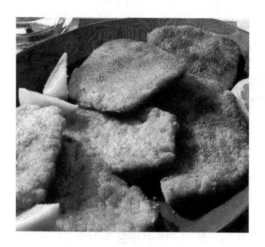

Total Time: 30 min | Prep: 20 min. Cook: 10 min. |
Makes: 4 servings

Ingredients

- 1/4 cup all-purpose flour
- 1 teaspoon prepared salt
- 1/4 teaspoon pepper
- 1 enormous egg
- 2 tablespoons 2% milk
- 3/4 cup dry bread scraps
- 1 teaspoon paprika
- 4 pork sirloin cutlets (4 ounces each)
- Cooking shower

DILL SAUCE:

- 1 tablespoon all-purpose flour
- 3/4 cup chicken stock
- 1/2 cup acrid cream
- 1/4 teaspoon dill weed

Directions

1. Preheat air fryer to 375°. In a shallow bowl, blend flour, prepared salt and pepper. In a subsequent shallow bowl, whisk egg and milk until mixed. In a third bowl, blend bread morsels and paprika.
2. Pound pork cutlets with a meat mallet to 1/4-in. thickness. Plunge cutlets in flour combination to cover the two sides; shake off abundance. Dunk in egg combination, at that point in piece blend, tapping to help covering follow.
3. Spot pork in a solitary layer on lubed plate in air-fryer bin; spritz with cooking splash. Cook until brilliant brown, 4-5 minutes. Turn; spritz with cooking splash. Cook until brilliant brown, 4-5 minutes longer. Eliminate to a serving plate; keep warm.
4. Then, in a small pot, whisk flour and stock until smooth. Heat to the point of boiling, mixing continually; cook and mix 2 minutes or until thickened. Diminish heat to low. Mix in harsh cream and dill; heat through (don't bubble). Present with pork.

30. Air-Fryer French Toast Cups with Raspberries

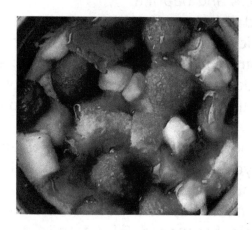

Total Time: 40 min | Prep: 20 min. + chilling Cook: 20 min. | Makes :2 servings

Ingredients
- 2 cuts Italian bread, cut into 1/2-inch 3D shapes
- 1/2 cup new or frozen raspberries
- 2 ounces cream cheddar, cut into 1/2-inch 3D shapes
- 2 huge eggs
- 1/2 cup entire milk
- 1 tablespoon maple syrup

RASPBERRY SYRUP:
- 2 teaspoons cornstarch
- 1/3 cup water
- 2 cups new or frozen raspberries, partitioned
- 1 tablespoon lemon juice

- 1 tablespoon maple syrup
- 1/2 teaspoon ground lemon zing
- Ground cinnamon, optional

Directions

1. Gap a large portion of the bread blocks between 2 lubed 8-oz. custard cups. Sprinkle with raspberries and cream cheddar. Top with residual bread. In a small bowl, whisk eggs, milk and syrup; pour over bread. Cover and refrigerate for at any rate 60 minutes.
2. Preheat air fryer to 325°. Spot custard cups on plate in air-fryer bin. Cook until brilliant brown and puffed, 12-15 minutes.
3. Then, in a small pot, join cornstarch and water until smooth. Add 1-1/2 cups raspberries, lemon juice, syrup and lemon zing. Heat to the point of boiling; diminish heat. Cook and mix until thickened, around 2 minutes. Strain and dispose of seeds; cool somewhat.
4. Tenderly mix staying 1/2 cup berries into syrup. Whenever wanted, sprinkle French toast cups with cinnamon; present with syrup.

31. Air-Fryer Raspberry Balsamic Smoked Pork Chops

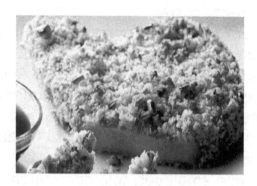

Total Time: 30 min | Prep: 15 min. Cook: 15 min./batch | Makes: 4 servings

Ingredients

- 2 large eggs
- 1/4 cup 2% milk
- 1 cup panko bread scraps
- 1 cup finely chopped walnuts
- 4 smoked bone-in pork cleaves (7-1/2 ounces each)
- 1/4 cup all-purpose flour
- Cooking shower
- 1/3 cup balsamic vinegar
- 2 tablespoons brown sugar
- 2 tablespoons seedless raspberry jam
- 1 tablespoon defrosted frozen squeezed orange concentrate

Directions

1. Preheat air fryer to 400°. In a shallow bowl, whisk together eggs and milk. In another shallow bowl, throw bread scraps with walnuts.
2. Coat pork cleaves with flour; shake off abundance. Dunk in egg blend, at that point in morsel combination, tapping to help follow. In groups, place hacks in single layer on lubed plate in air-fryer bushel; spritz with cooking splash.
3. Cook until brilliant brown and a thermometer embedded in pork peruses 145°, 12-15 minutes, turning part of the way through cooking and spritzing with extra cooking shower. In the mean time, place remaining ingredients in a small pot; heat to the point of boiling. Cook and mix until marginally thickened, 6-8 minutes. Present with cleaves.

32. Air-Fryer Green Tomato Stacks

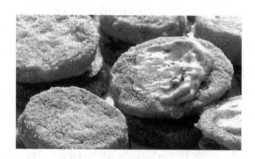

Total Time: 35 min | Prep: 20 min. Cook: 15 min./batch | Makes: 8 servings

Ingredients

- 1/4 cup without fat mayonnaise
- 1/4 teaspoon ground lime zing
- 2 tablespoons lime juice
- 1 teaspoon minced new thyme or 1/4 teaspoon dried thyme
- 1/2 teaspoon pepper, separated
- 1/4 cup all-purpose flour
- 2 huge egg whites, daintily beaten
- 3/4 cup cornmeal
- 1/4 teaspoon salt
- 2 medium green tomatoes
- 2 medium red tomatoes
- Cooking splash
- 8 cuts Canadian bacon, warmed

Directions

1. Preheat air fryer to 375°. Blend mayonnaise, lime zing and juice, thyme and 1/4 teaspoon pepper; refrigerate until serving. Spot flour in a shallow bowl; place egg whites in a different shallow bowl. In a third bowl, blend cornmeal, salt and staying 1/4 teaspoon pepper.
2. Cut every tomato transversely into 4 cuts. Daintily coat each cut in flour; shake off overabundance. Plunge in egg whites, at that point in cornmeal combination.
3. In clusters, place tomatoes on lubed plate in air-fryer container; spritz with cooking splash. Cook until brilliant brown, 4-6 minutes. Turn; spritz with cooking splash. Cook until brilliant brown, 4-6 minutes longer.
4. For each serving, stack 1 cut each green tomato, bacon and red tomato. Present with sauce.

33. Air-Fryer Papas Rellenas

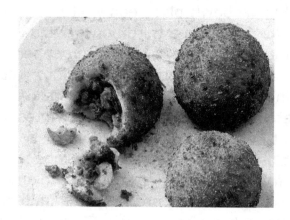

Total Time: 1 hr. | Prep: 45 min. Cook: 15 min./batch | Makes: 2-1/2 dozen

Ingredients
- 2-1/2 pounds potatoes (around 8 medium), stripped and cut into wedges
- 1 pound lean ground meat (90% lean)
- 1 small green pepper, finely chopped
- 1 small onion, finely chopped
- 1/2 cup pureed tomatoes
- 1/2 cup cut green olives with pimientos
- 1/2 cup raisins
- 1-1/4 teaspoons salt, partitioned
- 1-1/4 teaspoons pepper, partitioned
- 1/2 teaspoon paprika
- 1 teaspoon garlic powder
- 2 huge eggs, daintily beaten
- 1 cup prepared bread scraps
- Cooking splash

Directions

1. Spot potatoes in a huge pot and cover with water. Heat to the point of boiling. Lessen heat; cover and cook until delicate, 15-20 minutes.

2. In the meantime, in a huge skillet, cook hamburger, green pepper and onion over medium heat until meat is not, at this point pink; channel. Mix in pureed tomatoes, olives, raisins, 1/4 teaspoon salt, 1/4 teaspoon pepper and paprika; heat through.

3. Channel potatoes; squash with garlic powder and staying 1 teaspoon salt and pepper. Shape 2 tablespoons potatoes into a patty; place a storing tablespoon of filling in the middle. Shape potatoes around filling, framing a ball. Rehash.

4. Spot eggs and bread scraps in independent shallow dishes. Dunk potato balls in eggs, at that point move in bread morsels. Preheat air fryer to 400°. In clusters, place in single layer on lubed plate in air-fryer bushel; spritz with cooking shower. Cook until brilliant brown, 14-16 minutes.

34. Air-Fryer Nashville Hot Chicken

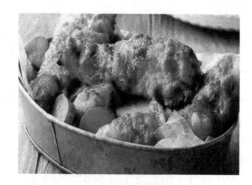

Total Time: 40 min | Prep: 30 min. Cook: 10 min. /batch | Makes: 6 servings

Ingredients
- 2 tablespoons dill pickle juice, partitioned
- 2 tablespoons hot pepper sauce, partitioned
- 1 teaspoon salt, separated
- 2 pounds chicken tenderloins
- 1 cup all-purpose flour
- 1/2 teaspoon pepper
- 1 huge egg
- 1/2 cup buttermilk
- Cooking splash
- 1/2 cup olive oil
- 2 tablespoons cayenne pepper
- 2 tablespoons dull brown sugar
- 1 teaspoon paprika
- 1 teaspoon stew powder
- 1/2 teaspoon garlic powder
- Dill pickle cuts

Directions

1. In a bowl or shallow dish, consolidate 1 tablespoon pickle juice, 1 tablespoon hot sauce and 1/2 teaspoon salt. Add chicken and go to cover. Refrigerate, covered, at any rate 60 minutes. Channel, disposing of any marinade.

2. Preheat air fryer to 375°. In a shallow bowl, blend flour, staying 1/2 teaspoon salt and the pepper. In another shallow bowl, whisk egg, buttermilk, and the leftover 1 tablespoon pickle juice and 1 tablespoon hot sauce. Dunk chicken in flour to cover the two sides; shake off overabundance. Dunk in egg blend, of course in flour combination.

3. In bunches, orchestrate chicken in a solitary layer on all around lubed plate in air-fryer container; spritz with cooking shower. Cook until brilliant brown, 5-6 minutes. Turn; spritz with cooking shower. Cook until brilliant brown, 5-6 minutes longer.

4. Whisk together oil, cayenne pepper, brown sugar and flavors; pour over hot chicken and throw to cover. Present with pickles.

35. Air-Fryer Mini Chimichangas

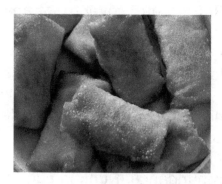

Prep: 1 hour Cook: 10 min. /batch | makes: 14 servings

Ingredients

- 1 pound ground hamburger
- 1 medium onion, chopped
- 1 envelope taco preparing
- 3/4 cup water
- 3 cups shredded Monterey Jack cheddar
- 1 cup acrid cream
- 1 can (4 ounces) chopped green chilies, depleted
- 14 egg move coverings
- 1 enormous egg white, gently beaten
- Cooking shower
- Salsa

Directions

1. In an enormous skillet, cook hamburger and onion over medium heat until meat is not, at this point pink; channel. Mix in taco preparing and water. Heat to the point of boiling. Lessen heat; stew, uncovered, for 5 minutes, blending occasionally. Eliminate from the heat; cool marginally.

2. Preheat air fryer to 375°. In an enormous bowl, join cheddar, acrid cream and chilies. Mix in meat blend. Spot an egg move covering on work surface with 1 point confronting you. Spot 1/3 cup filling in focus. Overlap base 33% of covering over filling; crease in sides.

3. Brush top point with egg white; move up to seal. Rehash with residual coverings and filling. (Continue to remain egg move coverings covered with waxed paper to abstain from drying out.)

4. In clumps, place chimichangas in a solitary layer on lubed plate in air-fryer container; spritz with cooking shower. Cook until brilliant brown, 3-4 minutes on each side. Serve warm with salsa and extra harsh cream.

36. Air-Fryer Loaded Pork Burritos

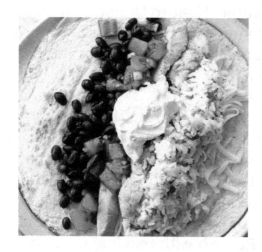

Total Time: 40 min | Prep: 35 min. + marinating
Cook: 5 min. | Makes: 6 servings

Ingredients

- 3/4 cup defrosted limeade concentrate
- 1 tablespoon olive oil
- 2 teaspoons salt, isolated
- 1-1/2 teaspoons pepper, separated
- 1-1/2 pounds boneless pork flank, cut into slim strips
- 1 cup chopped cultivated plum tomatoes
- 1 small green pepper, chopped
- 1 small onion, chopped
- 1/4 cup in addition to 1/3 cup minced new cilantro, separated
- 1 jalapeno pepper, cultivated and chopped
- 1 tablespoon lime juice
- 1/4 teaspoon garlic powder

- 1 cup uncooked long grain rice
- 3 cups shredded Monterey Jack cheddar
- 6 flour tortillas (12 inches), warmed
- 1 can (15 ounces) dark beans, washed and depleted
- 1-1/2 cups sharp cream
- Cooking splash

Directions

1. In a huge shallow dish, join the limeade concentrate, oil, 1 teaspoon salt and 1/2 teaspoon pepper; add pork. Go to cover; cover and refrigerate in any event 20 minutes.
2. For salsa, in a small bowl, join the tomatoes, green pepper, onion, 1/4 cup cilantro, jalapeno, lime juice, garlic powder and staying salt and pepper. Put in a safe spot.
3. Then, cook rice as per bundle directions. Mix in leftover cilantro; keep warm.
4. Channel pork, disposing of marinade. Preheat air fryer to 350°. In clusters, place pork in a solitary layer on lubed plate in air-fryer bushel; spritz with cooking splash. Cook until pork is not, at this point pink, 8-10 minutes, turning part of the way through.
5. Sprinkle 1/3 cup cheddar helter-skelter on every tortilla. Layer each with 1/4 cup salsa, 1/2 cup rice combination, 1/4 cup dark beans and 1/4 cup acrid cream, top with around 1/2 cup pork. Overlap sides and finishes over filling. Present with outstanding salsa.

37. Air-Fryer Beefy Swiss Bundles

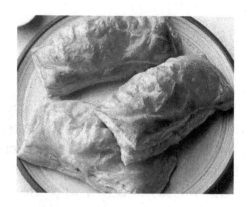

Total Time: 30 min | Prep: 20 min. Cook: 10 min. /batch | Makes: 4 servings

Ingredients

- 1 pound ground hamburger
- 1-1/2 cups cut new mushrooms
- 1/2 cup chopped onion
- 1-1/2 teaspoons minced garlic
- 4 teaspoons Worcestershire sauce
- 3/4 teaspoon dried rosemary, squashed
- 3/4 teaspoon paprika
- 1/2 teaspoon salt
- 1/4 teaspoon pepper
- 1 sheet frozen puff baked good, defrosted
- 2/3 cup refrigerated pureed potatoes
- 1 cup shredded Swiss cheddar
- 1 enormous egg
- 2 tablespoons water

Directions
1. Preheat air fryer to 375°. In an enormous skillet, cook hamburger, mushrooms and onion over medium heat until meat is not, at this point pink and vegetables are delicate, 8-10 minutes. Add garlic; cook brief longer. Channel. Mix in Worcestershire sauce and flavors. Eliminate from the heat; put in a safe spot.
2. On a delicately floured surface, fold puff baked good into a 15x13-in. square shape. Cut into four 7-1/2x6-1/2-in. square shapes. Spot around 2 tablespoons potatoes over every square shape; spread to inside 1 in. of edges. Top each with 3/4 cup hamburger combination; sprinkle with 1/4 cup cheddar.
3. Beat egg and water; brush some over baked good edges. Bring inverse corners of cake over each group; squeeze creases to seal. Brush with outstanding egg blend. In groups, place cakes in a solitary layer on plate in air-fryer bin; cook until brilliant brown, 10-12 minutes.
4. Freeze choice: Freeze unbaked cakes on a material lined heating sheet until firm. Move to an airtight compartment; get back to cooler. To utilize, cook frozen cakes as coordinated until brilliant brown and heated through, expanding time to 15-20 minutes.

Conclusion

I would like to thank you for choosing this book. Air frying is more grounded than fricasseeing in oil. It slices calories by 70% to 80% and has significantly less fat. This cooking strategy may likewise eliminate a portion of the other unsafe impacts of oil searing, All the recipes in this book are easy to prepare and will prove beneficial for beginners. Try these delicious recipes and appreciate!